# Copyright ©

GW00808309

1

## Table of Contents

## What Does the Current Research Say About Plant-Based Diets?

Most people who adopt this way of eating do it for the potential health benefits. "There have been many cardiac benefits linked to eating this way, like reduced cholesterol," Manaker says. "Some studies suggest that eating a plant-based diet may improve fertility parameters, and it also may reduce your risk of developing [type 2] diabetes."

One study linked diets rich in healthy plant foods (such as nuts, whole grains, fruits, veggies, and oils) with a significantly lower risk of heart disease.

Another study found it can also help prevent and treat type 2 diabetes, and it cites research that suggests this diet may help reduce the risk of other chronic illnesses, including cancer. (4)

# Food List of What to Eat, Limit, and Avoid

## What to Eat and Drink

• Vegetables (including kale, spinach, Swiss chard, collard greens, sweet potatoes, asparagus, bell peppers, and broccoli)

• Fruits (such as avocado, strawberries, blueberries, watermelon, apples, grapes, bananas, grapefruit, and oranges)

• Whole grains (such as quinoa, farro, brown rice, whole-wheat bread, and whole-wheat pasta)

• Nuts (walnuts, almonds, macadamia nuts, and cashews all count)

• Seeds (such as flaxseed, chia seeds, and hemp seeds)

• Beans

• Lentils

• Coffee

• Tea (including green, lavender, chamomile, or ginger)

What to Limit (or Avoid Entirely, Depending on How Strict You Decide to Be)

- Dairy (including milk and cheese)

- Meat and poultry (like chicken, beef, and pork)

- Processed animal meats, such as sausages and hot dogs

- All animal products (including eggs, dairy, and meat if you're following a vegan diet)

- Refined grains (such as "white" foods, like white pasta, rice, and bread)

- Sweets (like cookies, brownies, and cake)

- Sweetened beverages, such as soda, and fruit juice

- Potatoes and french fries

- Honey (if not vegan)

It is only until recently that more and more people are starting to embrace the plant-based diet lifestyle. As to what exactly has drawn tens of millions of people into this lifestyle is debatable. However, there is growing evidence demonstrating that following a primarily plant-based diet lifestyle leads to better weight control and general health, free of many chronic diseases.

Plant-based diets have gained popularity not only in the health and medical community, but also among fitness fanatics, athletes, and environmentalists. If you adopt the eating plan, you are likely to see improvement in the way you look or feel. But remember that the quality of your diet matters most.

A plant-based diet full of processed foods, added sugars, and sodium is probably not going to give you the results you desire. The best diet is a healthy diet that you can stick to for the long-term. Make gradual changes and enlist the help of a registered dietitian if necessary to put together a plan that keeps you healthy and satisfied.

# CHAPTER 1

## What Is A Plant-Based Diet

A lot of people are doing it; a lot of people are talking about it, but there is still a lot of confusion about what a whole food plant-based diet really means. Because we break food into its macronutrients: carbohydrates, proteins, and fats; most of us get confused about how to eat. What if we could put back together those macronutrients again so that you can free your mind of confusion and stress? Simplicity is the key here. Whole foods are unprocessed foods that come from the earth. Now, we do eat some minimally processed foods on a whole foods plant-based diet such as whole bread, whole wheat pasta, tofu, non-dairy milk and some nuts and seed butter. All these are fine as long as they are minimally processed. So, here are the different categories: Whole grains Legumes (basically lentils and beans) Fruits and vegetables Nuts and seeds (including nut butter) Herbs and spices All the above-mentioned categories make up a whole foods plant-based diet. Where the fun comes in is in how you prepare them; how you season and cook them; and how you mix and match to give them great flavor and variety in your meals.

As long as you are eating foods like these on a regular basis, you can forget about carbs, protein and fat forever. Now, some people might say, "well, I can't eat soy" or "I don't like tofu" and so on. Well, the beauty of a whole food plant based diet is that if you don't like a certain food, like in this case, soy, then you don't have to consume it. It is not a necessary component in a whole food plant-based diet. You can have brown rice instead of oats, quinoa instead of wheat; I'm sure you catch the drift now. It doesn't really matter. Just find something that suits you. Just because you have made the decision to adopt a plant-based diet lifestyle, doesn't mean that is a healthy diet. Plant-based diets have their fair share of junk and other unhealthy eats; case and point, regular consumption of veggie pizzas and non-dairy ice cream. Staying healthy requires you to eat healthy foods – even within a plant-based diet setting.

## Why You Need to Cut Back On Processed and Animal-Based Products

You've probably heard time and time again that processed food is bad for you. "Avoid preservatives; avoid processed foods"; however, no one ever really gives you any real or solid information on why you should avoid them and why they are dangerous. So let's break it down so that you can fully understand why you should avoid these culprits. They have huge addictive properties As humans, we really have a strong tendency to be addicted to certain foods, but the fact is that it's not entirely our fault. Practically all of the unhealthy eats we indulge in, from time to time, activate our brains dopamine neurotransmitter. This makes the brain feel "good" but only for a short period of time. This also creates an addiction tendency; that is why someone will always find themselves going back for another candy bar – even though they don't really need it. You can avoid all this by removing that stimulus altogether.

**They are loaded sugar and high fructose corn syrup**

Processed and animal-based products are loaded with sugars and high fructose corn syrup which have close to zero nutritional value. More and more studies are now proving what a lot of people suspected all along; that genetically modified foods cause gut inflammation which in turn makes it harder for the body to absorb essential nutrients. The downside of your body failing to properly absorb essential nutrients, from muscle loss and brain fog to fat gain, cannot be stressed enough.

They are loaded with refined carbohydrates

Processed foods and animal-based products are loaded with refined carbs. Yes, it is a fact that your body needs carbs to provide energy to run body functions. However, refining carbs eliminates the essential nutrients; in the way that refining whole grains eliminates the whole grain component. What you are left with after refining is what's referred to as "empty" carbs. These can have a negative impact on your metabolism by spiking your blood sugar and insulin levels.

**They are loaded with artificial ingredients**

When your body is consuming artificial ingredients, it treats them as a foreign object. They essentially become an invader. Your body isn't used to recognizing things like sucralose or these artificial sweeteners. So, your body does what it does best. It triggers an immune response which lowers your resistance making you vulnerable to diseases. The focus and energy spent by your body in protecting your immune system could otherwise be diverted elsewhere.

## They contain components that cause a hyper reward sense in your body

What this means is that they contain components like monosodium glutamate (MSG), components of high fructose corn syrup and certain dyes that can actually carve addictive properties. They stimulate your body to get a reward out of it. MSG, for instance, is in a lot of pre-packaged pastries. What this does is that it stimulates your taste buds to enjoy the taste. It becomes psychological just by the way your brain communicates with your taste buds. This reward-based system makes your body want more and more of it putting you at a serious risk of caloric overconsumption. What about animal protein? Often times the term "low quality" is thrown around to refer to plant proteins since they tend to have lower amounts of essential amino acids compared to animal protein. What most people do not realize is that more essential amino acids can be quite damaging to your health.

## Animal Protein Lacks Fiber

In their quest to load up on more animal protein most people end up displacing the plant protein that they already had. This is bad because unlike plant protein, animal protein often lacks in fiber, antioxidants, and phytonutrients. Fiber deficiency is quite common across different communities and societies in the world. In the USA, for instance, according to the Institute of Medicine, the average adult consumes just about 15 grams of fiber per day against the recommended 38 grams. Lack of adequate dietary fiber intake is associated with an increased risk of colon and breast cancers, as well as Crohn's disease, heart disease, and constipation.

## Animal protein causes a spike in IGF-1

IGF-1 is the hormone insulin-like growth factor-1. It stimulates cell division and growth, which may sound like a good thing but it also stimulates the growth of cancer cells. Higher blood levels of IGF-1 are thus associated with increased cancer risks, malignancy, and proliferation.

**Animal Protein causes an increase in Phosphorus**

Animal protein contains high levels of phosphorus. Our bodies normalize the high levels of phosphorus by secreting a hormone called fibroblast growth factor 23 (FGF23). This hormone has been found to be harmful to our blood vessels, thanks to a 2013 study titled, "Circulating Fibroblast Growth Factor 23 Is Associated with Angiographic Severity and Extent of Coronary Artery Disease". FGF23 has also been found to cause irregular enlargement of cardiac muscles – a risk factor for heart failure and even death in extreme cases. Given all the issues, the "high quality" aspect of animal protein might be more appropriately described as "high risk" instead. Unlike caffeine, which you will experience withdrawal once you cut it off completely, processed foods can be cut off instantaneously. Perhaps the one thing that you'll miss is the convenience of not having to prepare every meal from scratch.

## Plant-Based Diet vs. Vegan

It is quite common for people to mistake a vegan diet for a plant-based diet or vice versa. Well, even though both diets share similarities, they are not exactly the same. So let's break it down real quick.

# Vegan

A vegan diet is one that contains no animal-based products. This includes meat, dairy, eggs as well as animal-derived products or ingredients such as honey. Someone who describes themselves as a vegan carries over this perspective into their everyday life. What this means is that they do not use or promote the use of clothes, shoes, accessories, shampoo, and makeups that have been made using material that comes from animals. Examples here include wool, beeswax, leather, gelatin, silk, and lanolin. The motivation for people to lead a veganism lifestyle often stems from a desire to make a stand and fight against animal mistreatment and poor ethical treatment of animals as well as to promote animal rights.

## Plant Based Diet

 A whole food plant based diet in the other hand shares a similarity with veganism in the sense that it also does not promote dietary consumption of animal-based products. This includes dairy, meat, and eggs. What's more is that, unlike the vegan diet, processed foods, white flour, oils and refined sugars are not part of the diet. The idea here is to make a diet out of minimally processed to unprocessed fruits, veggies, whole grains, nuts, seeds, and legumes. So, there will be NO Oreo cookies for you. Whole-food plant-based diet followers are often driven by the health benefits it brings. It is a diet that has very little to do with restricting calories or counting macros but mostly to do with preventing and reversing illnesses.

## Getting Started on a Whole Food Plant-Based Diet

A common misconception among many people – even some of those in the health and fitness industry is that anyone who switches to a plant-based diet automatically becomes super healthy. There are tons of plant-based junk foods out there such as non-dairy ice cream and frozen veggie pizza, which can really derail your health goals if you are constantly consuming them. Committing to healthy foods the only way that you can achieve health benefits. On the other hand, these plant-based snacks do play a role in keeping you motivated. They should be consumed in moderation, sparingly and in small bits. As you will come to see later on in this book, there is a chapter dedicated to giving ideas on plant-based snacks you can whip up at home. So, without further ado, this is how you get started on a whole food plant-based recipe.

## Decide What a Plant-Based Diet Means

For You Making a decision to structure how your plant-based diet is going to look is the first step, and it is going to help you transition from your current diet outlook. This is something that is really personal and varies from one person to the other. While some people decide that they will not tolerate any animal products at all, some make do with tiny bits of dairy or meat occasionally. It is really up to you to decide what and how you want your plant-based diet to look like. The most important thing is that whole plant-based foods have to make a great majority of your diet.

## Understand What You Are Eating

All right, now that you've gotten the decision part down, your next task is going to involve a lot of analysis on your part. What do we mean by this? Well, if this is your first time trying out the plant-based diet, you may be surprised by the number of foods, especially packaged foods, which contain animal products. You will find yourself nurturing the habit of reading labels while you are shopping. Turns out, lots of prepackaged foods have animal products in them, so if you want to stick only to plant products for your new diet, you'll need to keep a keen eye on ingredient labels. Perhaps you decided to allow some amount of animal products in your diet; well, you are still going to have to watch out for foods loaded with fats, sugars, sodium, preservatives and other things that could potentially impact your healthy diet.

## Find Revamped Versions of Your Favorite Recipes

I'm sure you have a number of favorite dishes that are not necessarily plant-based. For most people, leaving all that behind is usually the hardest part. However, there is still a way you could meet halfway. Take some time to ponder what you like about those non-plant based meals. Think along the lines of flavor, texture, versatility and so on; and look for swaps in the whole food plant-based diet that can fulfill what you will be missing. Just to give you some insight into what I mean, here are a couple of examples: Crumbled or blended tofu would make for a decent filling in both sweet and savory dishes just like ricotta cheese would in lasagna. Lentils go particularly well with saucy dishes that are typically associated with meatloaf and Bolognese.

## Build a Support Network

Building any new habit is tough, but it doesn't have to be. Find yourself some friends, or even relatives, who are willing to lead this lifestyle with you. This will help you stay focused and motivated while also providing emotional support and some form of accountability. You can do fun stuff like trying out and sharing new recipes with these friends or even hitting up restaurants that offer a variety of plant-based options. You can even go a step further and look up local plantbased groups on social media to help you expand your knowledge and support network.

# CHAPTER 2

## The Benefits of Going Plant-Based

More and more people are becoming aware of the ability of a whole food plant based diet to help alleviate and even cure many chronic diseases such as heart disease, type 2 diabetes, arthritis, cancers, autoimmune disease, kidney stones, inflammatory bowel diseases and many more. Not to mention, a plant-based diet is more economical – especially when you buy local organic produce that is in season. So let's check out some of the benefits of going plant-based.

• It Lowers Blood Pressure:

Plant-based foods tend to have a higher amount of potassium whose benefits, notably include: reducing blood pressure and alleviating stress and anxiety. Some foods rich in potassium include legumes, nuts, seeds, whole grains, and fruits. Meat, on the other hand, contains very little to no potassium.

• It Lowers Cholesterol

Plants contain NO cholesterol – even the saturated sources like cacao and coconut. Leading a plant-based lifestyle will, therefore, help you lower the levels of cholesterol in your body leading to reduced risks of heart disease.

• Checks Your Blood Sugar Levels

Plant-based foods tend to have a lot of fiber. This helps slow down the absorption of sugars into the bloodstream as well as keep you feeling full for longer periods of time. It also helps balance out your blood cortisol levels thereby reducing stress.

• It Helps Prevent and Fight Off Chronic Diseases

In societies where a majority of people lead a plant-based lifestyle the rates of chronic diseases such as cancer, obesity, and diabetes are usually very low. This diet has also been proven to lengthen the lives of those already suffering from these chronic diseases.

• It Is Good for Weight Loss

Consuming whole plant-based foods make it easier to cut off excess weight and maintain a healthier weight without having to involve calorie restrictions. This is because Weight loss naturally occurs when you consume more fiber, vitamins, and minerals than you do animal fats and proteins.

## What to Look out For When Adopting this Lifestyle

For most people looking to go plant-based, protein is always a major concern. There is this notion that's perpetuated by the mainstream media backed by big meat producers that protein is only found in meat. Well, that's just not true. Traditional staples such as nuts, beans, oats and brown rice come with a lot of protein. Often times, nutrients like calcium are also marketed as coming from only animal-based sources. The truth is that foods like kale, broccoli, and almonds contain lots of calcium. Ask yourself this, if calcium comes from meat, then where did the animal get it from? It's definitely from the greens they eat.

The major concern for most plant-based diet followers is usually vitamin B12. B12, for everyone, is usually found in fortified products, especially cereals and plant-based milk.

However, those shouldn't be relied on to get enough of this important vitamin. The best option is to take a liquid or sublingual vitamin B12 supplement simply; just to make sure that there are no issues.

You can adopt a healthy plant-based lifestyle by basing your diet around cooked and raw foods filled with leafy and colorful veggies. These will provide your body with the minerals, vitamins, and antioxidants it needs

## A Quick word on Pantry Planning

As you transition into a whole-food, plant-based lifestyle, you don't have to worry about stocking. Your local farmer's market or grocery store should provide you with everything you need. Consider getting sets of transparent jars which you will use to store your food. This will make for a presentable look in your pantry. Typically, you will have some shelves dedicated to storage of grains, nuts, beans, spices, herbs and so on.

Stock Your Pantry

**Foods to Stock**

Non-Starchy Vegetables: Leafy greens (Kale, Spinach, Butter Lettuce etc.), Broccoli, Zucchini, Eggplant Tomatoes.

Starchy Vegetables: All kinds of potatoes, Whole corn, Legumes (all beans and lentils), Root vegetables, Quinoa

Fruits: All whole fruits (avoid dried and juiced fruits)

Whole Grains: 100% whole wheat, brown rice, and oats

Beverages: Water, Green tea, Unsweetened plant-based milk, Decaffeinated coffee and tea

Spices: All spices

Omega 3 Sources: Ground flax seed Chia seeds

Nuts Peanuts: Almonds, Cashews, Walnuts.

## Foods to Consume Sparingly

Avocadoes, Coconuts, Sesame seeds, Sunflower seeds, Pumpkin seeds, Dried fruit, Added sweeteners (maple syrup, fruit juice concentrate, and natural sugars), Caffeinated tea and coffee, Alcoholic beverages, Refined soy protein and wheat protein.

## Foods to Avoid

Meat: Fish, Poultry, Seafood, Red meat, Processed meat.

Dairy: Yogurt, Milk, Cheese, Cream, Half and half, Buttermilk.

Added Fats: Liquid oils, Coconut oil, Margarine, Butter.

Beverages: Soda, Fruit juice, Sports drinks, Energy drinks, Blended coffee and tea drinks

Refined Flours: All wheat flours that are not 100% whole wheat

Vegan Replacement Foods: Vegan "cheese" or vegan "meats" containing any oil

Miscellaneous: Eggs, Candy bars, Pastries, Cookies, Cakes, Energy bars

**A Quick Word on Labels**

When shopping to restock your pantry, always keep in mind that the goal is not to eat a lot of foods that require packaging or labels. However, it is normal to have that packaged food item on your list occasionally. When this does happen, these tips will help you stay vigilant and ensure a healthy shopping experience.

Do not believe company claims. Terms like 'low in fat' or '50% less sodium' are very popular on packaged foods. They don't really mean anything. What you should instead be focusing on is the ingredient list and the nutrition label. Just because a bag of potato chips has been labeled as having 40% less sodium doesn't mean that it is healthy. It could very well be still high in sodium or come with a host of other unwanted ingredients. The same goes for products labeled as "low-fat."

Make a habit of checking the ingredient. List As a general rule, the fewer ingredients there are, the healthier the food is. Such foods often have very few to no additives and preservatives which is good for your health. When you see the ingredients list containing a lot of words ending in "-ose," this is often an indicator that the food contains a lot of sugar. Also, check if there are any animal products on the ingredient list.

## Breakfast and Brunch Recipes

Maple Granola with Banana Whipped Topping

# Ingredients

2 cups of rolled oats

¼ cup of raw sunflower seeds

¼ cup of raw pumpkin seeds

¼ cup of raw unsweetened shredded dried coconut

¼ cup chopped walnuts

¼ cup raw or toasted wheat germ 1 teaspoon ground cinnamon

½ cup maple syrup

¾ cup raisins Banana Whipped Topping, optional

For Banana Whipped Topping

8 ounces soft or firm regular tofu, drained (sprouted variety is preferred)

1 ripe banana

2 tablespoons maple syrup, plus more as needed

## Instructions

i. Line a baking sheet with parchment paper and preheat your oven to 330 degrees F.

ii. Combine oats, pumpkin seeds, walnuts, sunflower seeds, cinnamon and wheat germ in a bowl along with maple syrup.

iii. Now in your baking sheet, spread the mixture evenly and bake for about 20 minutes.

iv. Stir in raisins and bake for another 5 minutes until the oats are golden.

v. Transfer to another baking sheet or tray and let it cool. You can serve it with banana toppings.

For Topping

Combine topping ingredients in a blender until smooth. Add maple syrup as desired.

**Chickpea Flour Scramble**

Ingredients

Chickpea flour batter:

½ cup of chickpea flour or use ½ cup + 1 or 2 tablespoons of more gram flour

½ cup of water

1 tablespoon of nutritional yeast

1 tablespoon of flaxseed meal

½ teaspoon of baking powder

¼ teaspoon of salt

¼ teaspoon of turmeric

¼ teaspoon or less paprika

1/8 teaspoon of Indian Sulphur black salt for the eggy flavor

Generous dash of black pepper

For Veggies:

1 teaspoon of oil divided

1 clove of garlic

¼ cup chopped onions

2 tablespoons each of asparagus green bell pepper, zucchini or other veggies.

½ green chili, chopped

2 tablespoons of chopped red bell pepper or tomato

Cilantro and black pepper for garnish

Instructions

i. Blend all the ingredients under chickpea flour batter and keep aside. You can also use lentil batter from my lentil frittata.

ii. Heat ½ teaspoon of oil in a skillet over medium heat. Add onion and garlic and cook for about 3 minutes until translucent.

iii. Add veggies, chili and cook for another 2 mins, then add spices and greens.

iv. Cover the veggies with the chickpea flour batter and continue cooking while adding olive oil.

v. Since the mixture tends to get doughy, be sure to scrap the bottom. Cook until the edges dry out. This should take about 5 minutes.

vi. Turn off the stove and break the food into smaller chunks then season with salt and pepper. You can garnish with cilantro if you like. Serve with toast or tacos.

# Peanut Butter and Jam Porridge

Ingredients

Peanut butter granola

½ cup of rolled oats or an assortment of cereals/nuts/seeds in your pantry

1 tablespoon peanut butter

1 teaspoon of rice malt syrup

Raspberry chia jam

¼ cup raspberries

1 tablespoon chia seeds

Porridge

⅔ Cup of rolled oats

1½  cup of coconut milk

2 tablespoon of peanut butter (optional)

1 banana, mashed (optional)

Other toppings

2 tablespoon of peanut butter

Whatever you desire! (Such as cacao nibs, coconut syrup, coconut and frozen berries)

Instructions

i. Preheat oven to 360°F.

ii. Combine granola ingredients in a baking sheet and bake for about 10 minutes (or until golden brown)

iii. Mash raspberries and mix in chia seeds then set it aside.

iv. Combine all porridge ingredients in a saucepan and bring to boil. Stir occasionally to maintain its smoothness.

v. Separate the porridge into 2 bowls and add granola, chia seeds, and peanut butter as desired.


**Banana Almond Granola**

Ingredients

8 cups rolled oats

2 cups pitted and chopped dates

2 ripe bananas, peeled and chopped

1 teaspoon almond extract

1 teaspoon salt

1 cup slivered almonds, toasted (optional)

Instructions

i. Preheat the oven to 275°F.

ii. Line a baking sheet with parchment paper.

iii. Cook dates covered with water in a saucepan over medium heat for about 10 minutes. Make sure the dates do not stick on the pan.

iv. Take the mixture off heat and in a blender, combine it with almond extract, bananas and salt until creamy.

v. Add oats to the date mixture and spread out on the baking sheet. Bake for about 45 minutes – occasionally stirring.

vi. Remove from oven and let it cool. Enjoy.

**Polenta with Pears and Cranberries**

Ingredients

¼ cup of brown rice syrup

2 pears, peeled, cored, and diced

1 cup of fresh or dried cranberries

1 teaspoon ground cinnamon

1 batch Basic Polenta, kept warm

Instructions

i. In a medium saucepan, combine the brown rice syrup, cranberries, pears and cinnamon. Cook until the pears are tender.

ii. Divide as desired and top with pear compote.

## Fruit and Nut Oatmeal

Ingredients

¾ cup of rolled oats

¼ teaspoon ground cinnamon Pinch of sea salt

¼ cup fresh berries (optional)

½ ripe banana, sliced (optional)

2 tablespoons of chopped nuts, such as walnuts, pecans, or cashews (optional)

2 tablespoons of dried fruit, such as raisins, cranberries, chopped apples, chopped Apricots (optional)

Maple syrup (optional)

Instructions

i. Cook oats in water in a saucepan until it starts boiling. Reduce the heat and let it simmer for about 5 minutes.

ii. Add cinnamon and salt – stirring. Top with berries and fruits and serve while hot.


Red Pesto and Kale Porridge

Ingredients

½ cup of oats

½ cup of couscous

2 cups of veggie stock (or water)

1 teaspoon of dried oregano

1 teaspoon of dried basil

1 cup of chopped kale

1 cup of sliced cherry tomatoes

1 scallion

1 teaspoon of tahini

1 tablespoon of pesto of your choice

2 tablespoons of nutritional yeast

1 tablespoon of pumpkin seed

1 tablespoon of hemp seed Salt and pepper to taste

Instructions

i. Cook oats, couscous, vegetable stock, oregano, basil, salt and pepper in a small pot on medium heat for about 5 minutes stirring occasionally.

ii. Once it becomes creamy, add scallions, chopped kale, and tomatoes. Stir in pesto, yeast, and tahini.

iii. Top with some cherry tomatoes hemp seeds and pumpkin and serve it warm.

**Spicy Tofu Scramble**

## Ingredients

350g of firm tofu

2 small spring onions, sliced

1 large garlic clove, finely chopped

10 cherry tomatoes, halved

½ fresh red chili, sliced

1 avocado, sliced

1 teaspoon of ground turmeric

2 teaspoon of ground black salt

Salt & pepper to taste

1 to 2 tablespoons of olive oil

8 slices of gluten-free bread, toasted


## Instructions

i. Sauté garlic in olive oil in a pan.

ii. Add in tomatoes and cook until they're soft then remove the mixture from the pan.

iii. Under a grill, toast bread slices. Sauté some onions and chili seeds on low-medium heat until they soften and add tofu.

iv. Sprinkle with turmeric and black salt and stir it for a couple of minutes. Finally, add tomatoes and garlic back to the pan to warm up.

v. Add the tofu scramble onto the toasted bread slices and decorate with avocado. Season as desired. Enjoy!

**Green Chia Pudding**

Ingredients

1 Medjool date with pit removed

1 cup non-dairy milk organic soy, almond, or coconut

1 handful fresh spinach

3 tablespoons of chia seeds

Fruit for topping banana, kiwi, mango or berries

Instructions

i. Combine the dates, milk, and spinach in a blender until smooth then add it to chia seeds in a medium bowl.

ii. Store in the refrigerator for up to overnight.

iii. Top with fruit before serving.

**Turmeric Steel Cut Oats**

Ingredients

¼ teaspoon of olive oil

½ cup of steel cut oats use certified gluten-free if needed

1½ cup of water 2 cups for a thinner consistency

1 cup of non-dairy milk

1/3 teaspoon of turmeric

½ teaspoon of cinnamon ¼ teaspoon of cardamom Salt to taste

2 tablespoons or more, of maple or other sweetener of your choice

Instructions

i. Toast oats in oil in a saucepan for a couple of minutes.

ii. Add water and milk and bring it to a boil before letting it simmer.

iii. Mix in the spices, salt, and maple and cook for about 8 minutes or until the oats are cooked to preference.

iv. Taste and adjust sweet, and flavors as desired then let it cool to thicken. You can serve warm or chilled.

v. Garnish with strawberries, dried fruit or chia seeds.

## Main Course Recipes

**Mashed Cauliflower and Green Bean Casserole**

Ingredients

¾ cup of coconut milk

½ cup of nutritional yeast

1 cauliflower Salt and pepper to taste

14 ounces of green beans, trimmed

1 onion, diced

## Instructions

i. In a skillet, cook cauliflower florets in vegetable broth and some olive oil.

ii. Add in onions and beans and cook for a little longer. Transfer the mixture into a blender and add coconut milk, nutritional yeast, salt and pepper and blend until smooth.

iii. In a baking sheet, assemble green bean mix, mashed cauliflower, and toppings and bake for 15 to 20 minutes at 400 degrees F. Enjoy.


**Zucchini Noodles with Portobello Bolognese**

Ingredients

3 tablespoons extra virgin olive oil, divided

6 Portobello mushroom caps, stems, and gills removed and finely chopped

½ cup of minced carrot

½ cup of minced celery

½ cup of minced yellow onion

3 large garlic cloves, minced

Kosher salt

Fresh ground pepper

1 tablespoon of tomato paste

A 28-ounce can crushed tomatoes (I strongly recommend San Marzano)

2 teaspoons of dried oregano

¼ teaspoon of crushed red pepper (optional)

½ cup fresh basil leaves, finely chopped (plus extra for serving)

4 medium zucchini

Instructions

i. Sauté garlic, mushrooms, celery, and carrots in olive oil in a pan. Season with salt and pepper as desired. Continue cooking until vegetables are soft.

ii. Stir in some tomato paste and cook for a couple of minutes before adding crushed tomatoes, oregano, red pepper, and basil.

iii. Let it simmer for 10 to 15 minutes until the sauce thickens. iv. As the sauce simmers, use an appropriate blade to make spiral zucchini.

v. Sauté the zucchini noodles in a separate saucepan for a couple of minutes and season as desired.

vi. Top with a generous amount of Bolognese and garnish with freshly chopped basil and serve immediately.

**Burrito Bowl**

Ingredients

Baked tortilla chips

2 to 4 cups cooked grains

2 to 4 cups cooked beans

2 to 4 cups chopped romaine lettuce or steamed kale

2 to 4 chopped tomatoes

1 to 2 chopped green onions

1 to 2 cups corn kernels

1 avocado, chopped

Fresh salsa

Instructions

i. Break some tortilla chips and place in a bowl.

ii. Add some cooked grains and beans.

 iii. Layer on tomatoes, lettuce, corn, onions, avocado and then top with salsa.

## Thai Noodles

Ingredients

8 ounces brown rice noodles or other whole-grain noodles

3 tablespoons of low-sodium soy sauce, or to taste

 2 tablespoons of brown rice syrup or maple syrup

2 tablespoons of fresh lime juice (from 1 to 2 limes)

4 garlic cloves, minced

3 cups of frozen Asian-style vegetables

1 cup of mung bean sprouts

2 green onions, white and light green parts chopped

3 tablespoons of chopped, roasted, unsalted peanuts

¼ cup of chopped fresh cilantro

1 lime, cut into wedges

Instructions

i. Follow instructions for cooking noodles.

ii. Combine soy sauce, garlic, brown rice syrup, lime juice and cup water and bring to a boil. Stir in the veggies and cook for about 5 minutes or until crisp-tender.

iii. Add the cooked noodles and mung bean sprouts and toss to coat then let it cook for a couple more minutes.

iv. Garnish with cilantro, green onions, lime wedges and chopped peanuts.

## Mediterranean Vegetable Spaghetti

Ingredients

10 ounces brown rice spaghetti

1 red bell pepper, cubed small

1 yellow bell pepper, cubed small

2 plum tomatoes, sliced into eighths (discard the seeds)
Salt

½ jalapeño (optional)

2 tablespoons of dried herbs de Provence

2 tablespoons of tomato purée

2 tablespoons apple cider vinegar or juice of 1 lime

12 cherry tomatoes, quartered

1 zucchini, halved then sliced into thin half-rounds

1 bunch spinach, chopped

Handful of black olives

## Instructions

i. Cook pasta, drain and set aside.

ii. Sauté peppers, tomatoes, jalapeno, and herbs in a saucepan. Add water and let it simmer.

iii. Add tomato puree and vinegar or lime juice and let it cook together for a few minutes until it becomes saucy.

iv. Add cherry tomatoes, zucchini slices, and spinach. Mix well and cook for about 5 to 7 minutes.

v. Add olives and sauce to the pasts along with some herbs. Enjoy

## Mexican Lentil Soup

Ingredients

2 tablespoons extra virgin olive oil

1 yellow onion, diced

2 carrots, peeled and diced

2 celery stalks, diced

1 red bell pepper, diced

3 cloves garlic, minced

1 tablespoon cumin

¼ teaspoon smoked paprika

1 teaspoon oregano

2 cups diced tomatoes and the juices

4 ounces diced green chilies

2 cups green lentils, rinsed and picked over

8 cups vegetable broth

½ teaspoon salt

A dash (or more) of hot sauce, plus more for serving

Fresh cilantro, for garnish

1 avocado, peeled, pitted, and diced, or garnish


Instructions

i. Sauté onions, celery, bell pepper and carrots in a pan for about 5 minutes then add garlic, cumin, paprika, and oregano and let it cook for another minute.

ii. Add in tomatoes, chilies, lentils, broth, and salt to taste and bring to a simmer until lentils are tender.

iii. Season with salt and pepper as necessary

iv. Serve it garnished with fresh cilantro, avocado, and a few dashes of hot sauce.

**Walnut Meat Tacos**

Ingredients

Walnut Tacos:

1½ cups de-shelled walnuts

1 teaspoon of garlic powder

½ teaspoon of cumin

½ teaspoon of chili powder

A tablespoon of tamari

6 Taco shells (organic & gluten-free)

Toppings:

1 cup carrots chopped

1 cup red cabbage chopped

¼ cup of onion, chopped

Cilantro chopped


Lime Cashew Sour Cream:

1 Cup cashews soaked overnight (or soaked at least 10 mins in boiling water)

½ cup of water (and more if needed)

2 tablespoons of lime juice

A tablespoon of apple cider vinegar

Pinch of salt to taste


Instructions

i. Blend walnuts in a food processor until it looks "meaty."

ii. Add walnuts to a food processor and process until mixture is kind of "meaty."

iii. Put mixture in a bowl and add seasonings and mix. Add the remaining ingredients and stir well.

iv. Fill taco shells with the mixture and top as desired.

v. Combine all ingredients of the lime cashew sour cream in a blender until smooth.

vi. Top tacos with sour cream and enjoy!

# DESSERT AND TREATS RECIPES

**Cream Decorated Truffles**

Ingredients

For the truffles:

2 tablespoons of organic raw cacao

½ cup of organic raw zucchini

½ cup of rolled oats

¼ cup Medjool dates or raisins

For the cream:

½ cup cashews

½ teaspoons of alcohol-free vanilla extract

2 Medjool dates, pitted

For decorating:

1 tablespoon filtered water

½ tsp. organic raw cacao

Instructions

i. Combine truffle ingredients in a blender until fully-fused.

ii. Using wet hands form the mixture into small balls and set aside.

iii. Combine cream ingredients in a blender until smooth then spread it over some of the truffles.

iv. Add two small pea size quantities of cream for the mummies' eyeballs for the remaining truffles.

v. Mix water and cacao in a small bowl and use a toothpick to make drops of the mixture onto the truffles. Enjoy


**Raw Apple Tart**

Ingredients

3 organic apples (of your choice), grated

A cup of dried cranberries

A cup of old-fashioned rolled oats

2 tablespoons of raw almond butter

1 cup of unsweetened coconut flakes

Instructions

i. Combine apples, cranberries, oats, and almond butter in a dish.

ii. Top with the coconut flakes, cover, and refrigerate for 2 hours.


## Raw Orange Chocolate Pudding

Ingredients

1 vanilla bean, seeds scraped out (or 1 ½ tsp pure vanilla extract)

A cup of peeled, pitted, and roughly chopped ripe avocado

1 cup pitted dates 1/3 cup raw or regular cocoa powder

1 teaspoon of orange zest

½ cup of freshly squeezed orange juice

1/8 teaspoon of sea salt

Instructions

i. Combine all ingredients in a food processor and puree until smooth.

ii. You can thin the puree by adding more orange juice, or a splash of nut milk or water.

iii. Serve or store in the refrigerator.

**Mango Chia Seed Pudding**

Ingredients

2 cups of coconut milk

½ cup of chia seeds

1 teaspoon of vanilla (powder or extract)

¼ teaspoon of cardamom

1 medium sized mango

3 tablespoons of coconut nectar or 2 tablespoons of date paste

Instructions

i. Mix chia seeds with coconut milk, coconut nectar, vanilla, and cardamom in a bowl and refrigerate up to overnight.

ii. Slice the mango up into pieces and puree in a blender.

iii. Serve accordingly – mix together or serve in layers and enjoy!


## Chewy Lemon and Oatmeal Cookies

Ingredients

10 dates, pitted

A cup of unsweetened applesauce

1½ teaspoons of apple cider vinegar

A cup of rolled oats A cup of oat flour

½ cup quick-cooking oats

¾ cup roughly chopped walnuts

2 tablespoons of grated lemon zest (from about 2 lemons)

2 teaspoons of natural cocoa powder

1 teaspoon of vanilla powder

½ teaspoon of baking soda

Pinch of sea salt to taste

## Instructions

i. Preheat the oven to 275°F and line 2 baking sheets with parchment paper.

ii. Soak the dates in hot water for about 20 minutes then blend them with applesauce and vinegar.

iii. Stir together the rolled oats, oat flour, quick-cooking oats, walnuts, lemon zest, cocoa powder, vanilla powder, baking soda, and salt in a large bowl.

iv. Mix in the dates and applesauce paste and make sure that the mixture is relatively dry.

v. Scoop a portion, roll it into a ball, pat it flat and place onto a baking sheet. Repeat this until you use up all the mixture.

vi. Bake for about 40 minutes until the tops of the cookies appear crispy and browned.

vii. Let them cool on a wire rack. Enjoy

## Chocolate Buckwheat Granola Bars

Ingredients

2 bananas

¼ cup of peanut butter (or almond butter)

1 tablespoon of cocoa powder

1 teaspoon of all-natural vanilla extract (I used my homemade one)

3 tablespoons of date syrup or maple syrup

1⅓ cup of buckwheat groats

⅓ - ½ cup of dark chocolate chunks (sweetened with healthy sweeteners if you can find it or you can use unsweetened and increase the date syrup by 1 tablespoon)

Instructions

i. Preheat the oven to 360 degrees F (180 degrees Celsius).

ii. Combine and mash the bananas with peanut butter, cocoa powder, vanilla extract and date syrup in a bowl.

iii. Add chocolate and buckwheat groats and pour into a brownie pan.

iv. Bake for about 20 minutes until the granola bars firm up then set it aside to cool. Enjoy

## Drinks and Smoothies Recipes

### Red Velvet Cake Smoothie

Ingredients

2 ripe bananas, peeled

½ medium beet, scrubbed and roughly chopped

½ cup of walnut pieces 4 to 6 pitted dates, depending on how sweet you want it

1 cup fresh packed spinach

¼ cup of unsweetened cocoa powder

1 teaspoon of pure vanilla extract

1½ cups of non-dairy milk such as almond, rice, or coconut

2 cups of ice

Optional Garnish:

Finely chopped dark chocolate

Finely chopped walnuts

Coconut flakes

Instructions

i. Combine all ingredients in a blender until a smoothie consistency is achieved.

ii. Garnish as desired and serve!

**Berry Soft Serve**

Ingredients

A large banana

¾ cup of frozen mixed berries

½ cup of nondairy milk

Instructions

i. The previous night: peel banana, break into chunks, and freeze

ii. Combine frozen banana, berries, and milk in a blender and blend until creamy and thick. Add a splash of milk to thin.

iii. Serve with some vegan brownies!

**Quinoa, Berry and Coconut Smoothie**

Ingredients

A cup of almond or coconut milk

A cup of raspberries

1 Medjool date

½ cup of cooked quinoa

2 tablespoons of dried goji berries

2 tablespoons of shredded coconut

Instructions

i. Remove the pit and put the date into your blender jar. Add in the rest of the ingredients

ii. Blend for until smooth. Refrigerate or drink right away.

Adopting a Whole-Foods, Plant-Based Diet Is Good for the Planet

Switching to a plant-based diet not only benefits your health — it can help protect the environment, as well.

People who follow plant-based diets tend to have smaller environmental footprints.

Adopting sustainable eating habits can help reduce greenhouse gas emissions, water consumption and land used for factory farming, which are all factors in global warming and environmental degradation.

A review of 63 studies showed that the largest environmental benefits were seen from diets containing the least amount of animal-based foods such as vegan, vegetarian and pescatarian diets.

The study reported that a 70% reduction in greenhouse gas emissions and land use and 50% less water use could be achieved by shifting Western diet patterns to more sustainable, plant-based dietary patterns.

What's more, reducing the number of animal products in your diet and purchasing local, sustainable produce helps drive the local economy and reduces reliance on factory farming, an unsustainable method of food production.

Foods to Eat on a Whole-Foods, Plant-Based Diet

From eggs and bacon for breakfast to steak for dinner, animal products are the focus of most meals for many people.

When switching to a plant-based diet, meals should center around plant-based foods.

If animal foods are eaten, they should be eaten in smaller quantities, with attention paid to the quality of the item.

Foods like dairy, eggs, poultry, meat and seafood should be used more as a complement to a plant-based meal, not as the main focal point.

# A Whole-Foods, Plant-Based Shopping List

• Fruits: Berries, citrus fruits, pears, peaches, pineapple, bananas, etc.

• Vegetables: Kale, spinach, tomatoes, broccoli, cauliflower, carrots, asparagus, peppers, etc.

• Starchy vegetables: Potatoes, sweet potatoes, butternut squash, etc.

• Whole grains: Brown rice, rolled oats, farro, quinoa, brown rice pasta, barley, etc.

• Healthy fats: Avocados, olive oil, coconut oil, unsweetened coconut, etc.

• Legumes: Peas, chickpeas, lentils, peanuts, black beans, etc.

• Seeds, nuts and nut butters: Almonds, cashews, macadamia nuts, pumpkin seeds, sunflower seeds, natural peanut butter, tahini, etc.

• Unsweetened plant-based milks: Coconut milk, almond milk, cashew milk, etc.

• Spices, herbs and seasonings: Basil, rosemary, turmeric, curry, black pepper, salt, etc.

• Condiments: Salsa, mustard, nutritional yeast, soy sauce, vinegar, lemon juice, etc.

• Plant-based protein: Tofu, tempeh, plant-based protein sources or powders with no added sugar or artificial ingredients.

• Beverages: Coffee, tea, sparkling water, etc.

If supplementing your plant-based diet with animal products, choose quality products from grocery stores or, better yet, purchase them from local farms.

• Eggs: Pasture-raised when possible.

• Poultry: Free-range, organic when possible.

• Beef and pork: Pastured or grass-fed when possible.

• Seafood: Wild-caught from sustainable fisheries when possible.

• Dairy: Organic dairy products from pasture-raised animals whenever possible.

## Foods to Avoid or Minimize on This Diet

The WFPB diet is a way of eating that focuses on consuming foods in their most natural form. This means that heavily processed foods are excluded.

When purchasing groceries, focus on fresh foods and, when purchasing foods with a label, aim for items with the fewest possible ingredients.

## Foods to Avoid

• Fast food: French fries, cheeseburgers, hot dogs, chicken nuggets, etc.

• Added sugars and sweets: Table sugar, soda, juice, pastries, cookies, candy, sweet tea, sugary cereals, etc.

• Refined grains: White rice, white pasta, white bread, bagels, etc.

• Packaged and convenience foods: Chips, crackers, cereal bars, frozen dinners, etc.

• Processed vegan-friendly foods: Plant-based meats like Tofurkey, faux cheeses, vegan butters, etc.

• Artificial sweeteners: Equal, Splenda, Sweet'N Low, etc.

- Processed animal products: Bacon, lunch meats, sausage, beef jerky, etc.

## Foods to Minimize

While healthy animal foods can be included in a WFPB diet, the following products should be minimized in all plant-based diets.

- Beef

- Pork

- Sheep

- Game meats

- Poultry

- Eggs

- Dairy

- Seafood

## A Sample Meal Plan for One Week

Transitioning to a whole-foods, plant-based diet doesn't have to be challenging.

The following one-week menu can help set you up for success. It includes a small number of animal products, but the extent to which you include animal foods in your diet is up to you.

Monday

• Breakfast: Oatmeal made with coconut milk topped with berries, coconut and walnuts.

• Lunch: Large salad topped with fresh vegetables, chickpeas, avocado, pumpkin seeds and goat cheese.

• Dinner: Butternut squash curry.

Tuesday

• Breakfast: Full-fat plain yogurt topped with sliced strawberries, unsweetened coconut and pumpkin seeds.

• Lunch: Meatless chili.

• Dinner: Sweet potato and black bean tacos.

Wednesday

• Breakfast: A smoothie made with unsweetened coconut milk, berries, peanut butter and unsweetened plant-based protein powder.

- Lunch: Hummus and veggie wrap.

- Dinner: Zucchini noodles tossed in pesto with chicken meatballs.

Thursday

- Breakfast: Savory oatmeal with avocado, salsa and black beans.

- Lunch: Quinoa, veggie and feta salad.

- Dinner: Grilled fish with roasted sweet potatoes and broccoli.

Friday

- Breakfast: Tofu and vegetable frittata.

- Lunch: Large salad topped with grilled shrimp.

- Dinner: Roasted portobello fajitas.

Saturday

- Breakfast: Blackberry, kale, cashew butter and coconut protein smoothie.

- Lunch: Vegetable, avocado and brown rice sushi with a seaweed salad.

• Dinner: Eggplant lasagna made with cheese and a large green salad.

Sunday

• Breakfast: Vegetable omelet made with eggs.

• Lunch: Roasted vegetable and tahini quinoa bowl.

• Dinner: Black bean burgers served on a large salad with sliced avocado.

As you can see, the idea of a whole-foods, plant-based diet is to use animal products sparingly.

However, many people following WFPB diets eat more or fewer animal products depending on their specific dietary needs and preferences.

**Recommended Timing**

There is no fasting required or special meal timing for following a WFPB diet. Some people who are trying to lose weight on a WFPB diet choose to limit carbs after dinner or eat only raw food until 4 p.m.

## Resources and Tips

If you are new to the WFPB lifestyle, there's no need to be intimidated as meatless diets are easier to follow than ever. The key is to stock your kitchen with healthy plant-based foods so you don't feel deprived.

• Take it one step at a time: If you're not sure if you're ready for the full commitment, take small steps to eat less meat. Take advantage of Meatless Mondays or challenge yourself to eat two to three meals each week that do not include meat or dairy.

• Make healthy swaps: You can still eat almost all of your favorite foods when you follow a WFPB diet. You just have to make a few clever swaps. Love burgers? Grill a portobello mushroom and place it on a bun with your favorite toppings. Enjoy pizza with a whole-wheat crust and colorful veggies instead of meat and cheese.

• Learn to love legumes: Beans are your friends on a WFPB program. Legumes provide protein and fiber which gives you the sense of fullness and satiety that you may have enjoyed when you ate meat. Stock up on a variety of canned or dried beans.

• Save money with frozen and bulk foods: Plant-based eating doesn't have to be expensive. Fresh fruits and vegetables are flavorful and have the best texture. But frozen foods are usually just as nutritious. Keep frozen berries, peas, corn, and other veggies on hand to throw into recipes. Buy seeds and nuts in bulk to save money.

## Pros and Cons

For the many health benefits of a WFPB diet, there are a few downsides. Like any whole-food diet, avoiding processed foods requires more meal planning and preparation than pre-packaged foods.

In addition, not eating meat can make it tricky to get enough protein and certain nutrients. Although, with careful planning and attention, nutritionists say you can get most of the nutrients you need from plants.

Pros

• Improved heart health

• Reduced risk of diabetes and diabetic complications

• Reduced risk of cancer

- Lower Body Mass Index (BMI)

- Wide variety of foods

- No weighing or measuring

Cons

- Difficult to ensure enough protein

- Possible nutrient deficiencies including calcium, iron, and B12

- Meal planning and preparation

Pros

A plant-based diet—in particular, one focused on whole, unprocessed foods—offers many health benefits, including improved heart health and decreased risks of diabetes, cancer, and obesity.

Many people following this way of eating report more energy, fewer aches and pains, and an overall sense of well-being.

Research shows that following a WFPB diet can be an effective weight-loss strategy. A 2016 meta-analysis of more than 1,151 subjects found individuals assigned to the vegetarian diet groups lost significantly more weight than those assigned to the non-vegetarian diet groups.

Additional research suggests the diet is effective for weight loss without needing to restrict calories, measure portions, or exercise.

While following a whole-foods, plant-based diet is considered a healthy way to eat, simply following a plant-based or vegetarian diet often includes processed foods that are not healthy. Without proper planning, it can be difficult to get enough protein and other nutrients needed for good health.

Cons

The biggest challenge of following a WFPB diet is making sure you get enough of key nutrients. People on vegetarian diets need to pay extra attention to ensure they get enough protein, calcium, iron, and vitamin B12.

According to the Academy of Nutrition and Dietetics, a well-planned plant-based diet can provide adequate nutrition. Vegetarian diets may lead to a reduced intake of certain nutrients, the report states, but deficiencies can be avoided by appropriate planning.10

## Protein

Protein is made up of a chain of amino acids, which the body needs in certain proportions to utilize the protein.

Amino acids are found in meats, milk, fish, eggs, nuts, legumes and grains. Animal products are a complete protein source because they contain all the necessary amino acids. Plant-based protein, however, is incomplete.

In the past, it was believed that in order for the body to utilize the amino acids in plants, foods need to be eaten in the right combination, for example, beans and rice.

However, in 2016 the Academy of Nutrition and Dietetics updated its recommendations to state that protein from a variety of plant foods eaten throughout the day works together to supply enough amino acids. In addition, the regular consumption of legumes and soy products will ensure adequate protein intake.10

## Iron

While people following a plant-based diet have similar iron intakes as meat eaters, vegetarians typically have lower blood levels of iron. This is because plant-based iron (or non-heme iron) is not as bioavailable as animal-based heme iron.

Due to this, the Institute of Medicine recommends people following a vegetarian diet aim to consume additional dietary iron and have iron levels monitored by a doctor. Taking iron supplements is not recommended unless advised by your doctor.11

Calcium

Getting enough calcium can also be difficult on a plant-based diet. While many vegetables are high in calcium, other components in plants—namely oxalate, phytate, and fiber—block their bioavailability.

Nutritionists recommend eating low-oxalate vegetables, such as kale, turnip greens, Chinese cabbage, and bok choy, calcium-set tofu (made with a calcium salt), and fortified plant milk, like almond or soy milk.10

Vitamin B12

Plants do not contain vitamin B12, which is needed for healthy blood cells and energy. People who follow a plant-based diet are unlikely to get adequate vitamin B12 without eating foods fortified in B12, such as breakfast cereals and nutritional yeast, or taking a B12 supplement.10 The recommended daily amount of B12 for adults is 2.4 mcg.12

How It Compares

The WFPB diet contains a wide variety of nutritious foods. With proper planning, it is possible to get all the necessary vitamins and nutrients with this way of eating.

However, many people following a plant-based diet that is not based on whole foods may end up eating unhealthy processed foods, which do not provide proper nutrition.

USDA Recommendations

The U.S. Department of Agriculture (USDA) dietary guidelines include calorie recommendations and tips for a healthy, balanced diet. The following nutrient-dense foods are recommended as part of a healthy diet:

• Vegetables and dark, leafy greens (kale, spinach, broccoli, Swiss chard, green beans)

• Fruits (apples, berries, melon)

- Grains (quinoa, brown rice, oats)

- Lean meats (chicken breast, fish, turkey breast)

- Beans and legumes (all beans, lentils, peas)

- Nuts and seeds (walnuts, almonds, sunflower seeds)

- Dairy (reduced fat milk, cheese, yogurt)

- Oils (olive oil, avocado oil)

Due to the elimination of meat and dairy, a plant-based diet does not meet the USDA guidelines, however, with proper planning, it is possible to get all the necessary nutrients through plants or with dietary supplements.

The USDA recommends consuming roughly 1,500 calories per day for weight loss, but this number varies based on age, sex, weight, and activity level.

Similar Diets

There are several variations of plant-based diets and some allow for animal products. Common plant-based diets include:

- Vegetarian diet: This plan avoids meat, seafood, and poultry, but eggs and dairy may be eaten (lacto-ovo vegetarians). People would not necessarily be considered plant-based eaters unless they limit their consumption.

• Vegan diet: On this diet, you avoid meat, seafood, poultry, eggs, and dairy products or any food made with those ingredients. The diet does not restrict processed foods, added sugars, or fat. It does not require the consumption of whole foods.

• Mediterranean diet: This diet emphasizes plant-based eating but encourages consumption of fish and allows for small amounts of chicken, dairy products, eggs, and red meat.

• Flexitarian diet: Also known as a "flexible vegetarian" diet, this eating plan emphasizes plant-based foods but allows for occasional allowances of foods that are not typically considered vegetarian.

• Raw food diet: Usually a vegan diet, you'd avoid all foods that you avoid on the vegan eating plan along with any foods cooked at temperatures greater than 118 degrees F.

• Fruitarian diet: This comprises a vegan diet that is mostly fruit.

• Macrobiotic diet: This is usually a vegan diet that emphasizes natural, organic whole foods that are grown locally. Plant-based foods are emphasized, but meat and seafood may be consumed occasionally.

Tips for Lazy Days and Dining Out

We all know that eating out can sometimes be challenging when you are following a whole food, plant-based diet and avoiding oil and other concentrated ingredients or if you need to eat gluten-free. On the other hand, ordering takeout or dine-in can be quite convenient after a long, hectic day where prepping food was simply not in your plans. So, here are some tips you can use when dining out.

i. Look up niche restaurants such as plant-based restaurants or vegan restaurants

ii. Specify how you want your meals prepared. Always opt for steamed, baked, water sautéed or grilled

iii. Play nice with the wait staff to get them to make your preferences happen.

# Conclusion

A whole-foods, plant-based diet is a way of eating that celebrates plant foods and cuts out unhealthy items like added sugars and refined grains.

Plant-based diets have been linked to a number of health benefits, including reducing your risk of heart disease, certain cancers, obesity, diabetes and cognitive decline.

Plus, transitioning to a more plant-based diet is an excellent choice for the planet.

Regardless of the type of whole-foods, plant-based diet you choose, adopting this way of eating is sure to boost your health.

Lightning Source UK Ltd.
Milton Keynes UK
UKHW010829010821
387995UK00001B/119